Sense of Self

Coping Skills For Kids
WORKBOOK

EASY TO READ INSTRUCTIONS
QUESTIONS AND ACTIVITIES
WORKSHEETS INCLUDED

by Sally Safadi

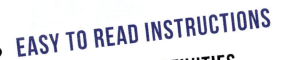

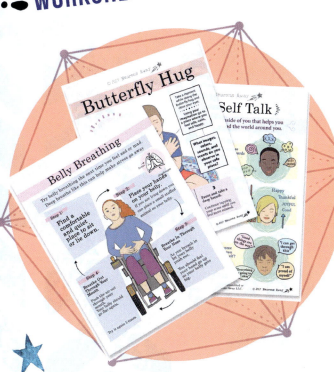

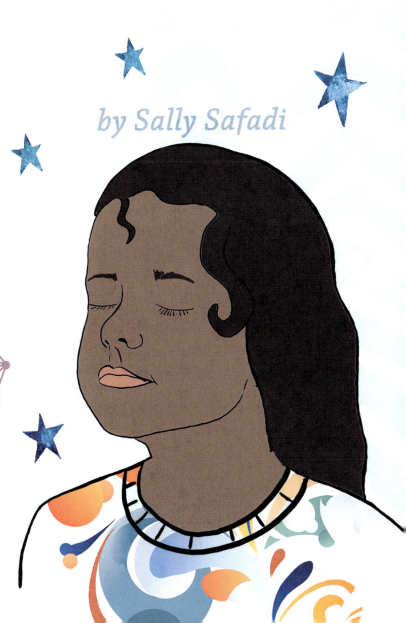

SENSE OF SELF
Coping Skills and Stress Management Tools for Kids

Written and Created by Sally Safadi

Published by Neurons Away LLC
Syracuse, New York
Copyright © 2020 Neurons Away

Hello!

This vibrant series focuses on the effectiveness and success of various coping and life skills. The workbook includes easy to read instructions, questions and activities that draw from DBT, CBT, educational theories and self-care practices.

The worksheets are only intended as supplemental tools to your practice and do not need to be done in any specific order. Just pick and choose whatever you'd like to work on.

You may use the material for personal use and small group use. If you wish to utilize the material with large groups or for commerical use please contact sally@neuronsaway.com.

Large sized posters that can be used in classrooms or therapy spaces can be purchased at **neuronsaway.com**

Thank you very much for your support! If you have any suggestions or would like to see a new coping skill added to the collection please reach out.

Have a great day!

{ Breathing }

Breathing is the process of bringing air in and out of the lungs. When you are feeling overwhelemed with emotions you can guide your breathing to make you feel better.

Breathing is simple, free, and with you at all times.

Easy Deep Breathing Exercise

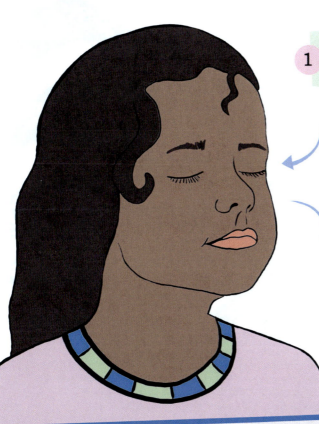

1 **Breathe in through your nose for 3 counts**
(while <u>breathing in</u> count 1..2..3..)

2 **Hold your breath for 3 counts**
(while <u>holding</u> your breath count 1..2..3..)

3 **Exhale through your mouth for 3 counts**
(while <u>breathing out</u> count 1..2..3...)

*Repeat 3 times!

How does deep breathing help?

-Helps clear your thoughts
-Helps calm your emotions
-Helps heal your body and mind

"A healthy mind has an easy breath."

{ Breathing is one of the greatest pleasures in life. }

Easy Deep Breathing Activity

1. Inhale through the nose for 3 counts
(while breathing in count 1..2..3..)

what do you want to bring in?

2. Hold your breath for 3 counts
(while holding your breath count 1..2..3..4..)

what do you want to hold within you?

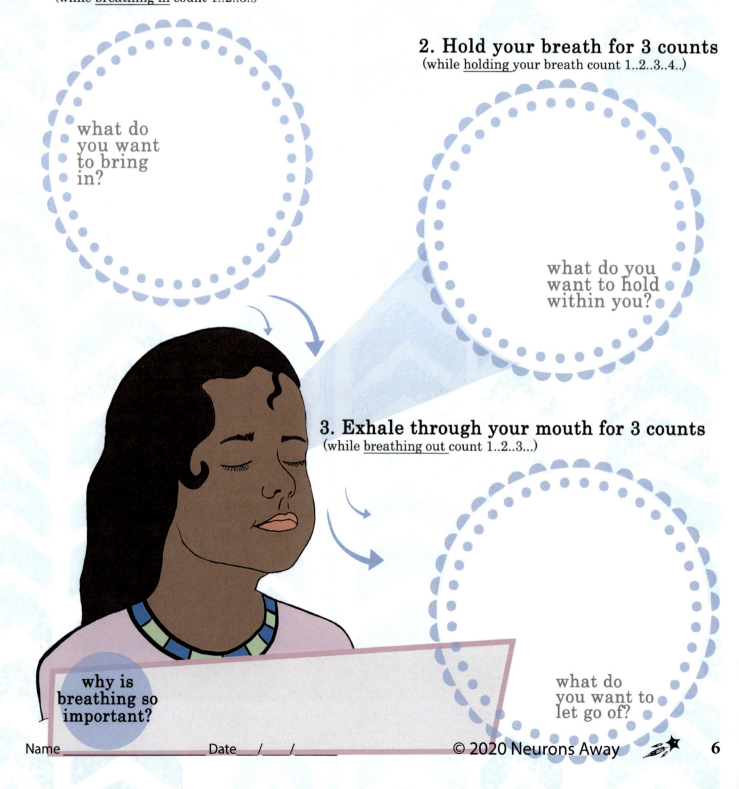

3. Exhale through your mouth for 3 counts
(while breathing out count 1..2..3...)

why is breathing so important?

what do you want to let go of?

Name_____ Date____/____/____

Belly Breathing

Try belly breathing the next time you feel sad or mad. Deep breaths like this can help make stress go away.

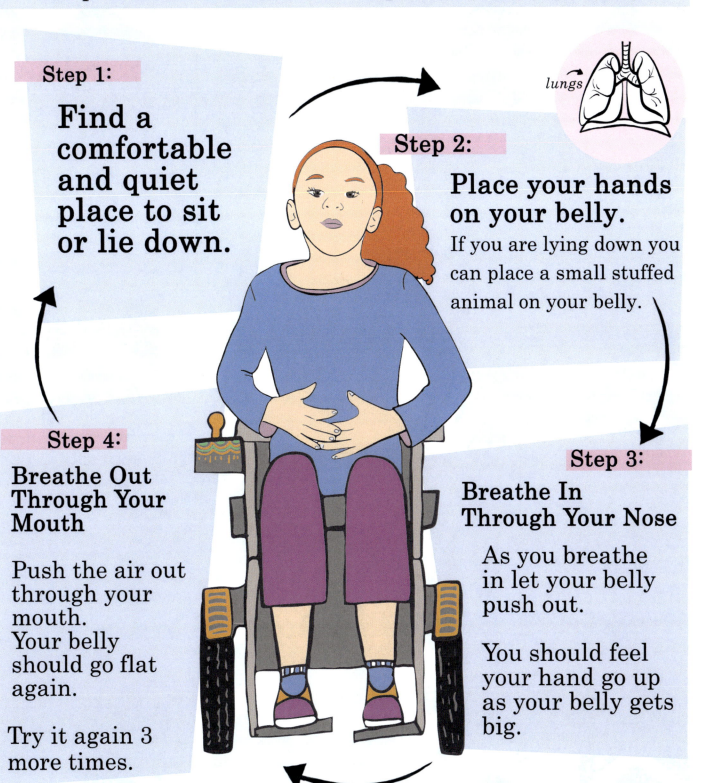

Step 1:

Find a comfortable and quiet place to sit or lie down.

lungs

Step 2:

Place your hands on your belly.

If you are lying down you can place a small stuffed animal on your belly.

Step 4:

Breathe Out Through Your Mouth

Push the air out through your mouth. Your belly should go flat again.

Try it again 3 more times.

Step 3:

Breathe In Through Your Nose

As you breathe in let your belly push out.

You should feel your hand go up as your belly gets big.

Name _____ Date___/___/_____

Butterfly Hug

Calm and sooth yourself with the butterfly hug when you are feeling sad, angry or hurt.

Take a moment while doing the butterfly hug and close your eyes.
· · · · · · · ·
Using your imagination go to a place where you feel safe, calm, and happy.

What images, colors, sounds, and scents do you observe in your safe place?

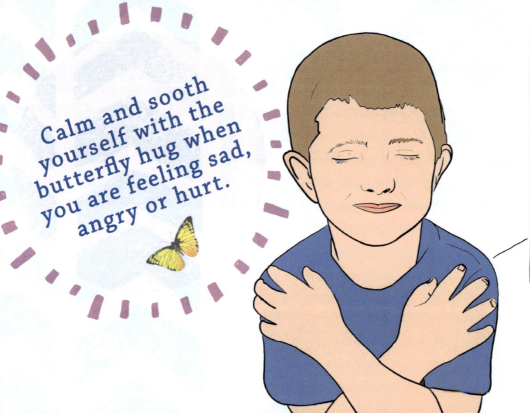

PRACTICE SELF-SOOTHING

1

Cross both arms over your chest and place each hand on your shoulder.

Breathe.

2

Gently begin tapping each hand one at a time on your arms.

Tap for 10 counts.

3

Pause and take a deep breath.

Continue tapping your arms until you feel more relaxed.

Butterfly Hug

Draw a place where you feel safe, calm, and content.

What colors, sounds, and scents do you observe in your safe place?

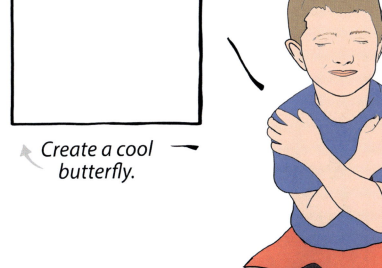

Create a cool butterfly.

Take a moment while doing the butterfly hug and close your eyes.

Name _____ Date____/____/_____

Meditation

Meditation is like taking a multivitamin for your health. It is great to do every day.

Benefits:
- Good for your body and mind
- Helps you make good decisions
- Helps you focus and pay attention
- Reduces panic and stress

1

Use your inner voice to prepare for meditation by repeating helpful sentences such as:

→ *"I am creating a safe space."*

→ *"I am happy, healthy and whole."*

→ *"I am safe and sound. All is well."*

2

Get in a comfortable position in a quiet space.

Examples:
- Sit up right in a chair
- Lay down on a bed
- Sit cross-legged on the ground

3

FOCUS ON YOUR BREATH
- Feel the air enter your nose
- Feel your lungs fill up with air
- Feel the air leaving your nose or mouth.

Start with 4 breaths work your way up to more.

4

Close your eyes and clear your mind
- Smile softly, feel it.
- Listen to your natural breathing
- Observe your heartbeat

TIPS:
- ★ Listen to calming music or a guided meditation
- ★ Softly hum a tune or repeat a mantra
- ★ Write in a journal before and after meditating
- ★ Create a space with items or pictures you admire.

Name_____ Date___/___/_____

Meditation

How do you think meditation will help you?

Benefits:

Meditation is like taking a multivitamin for your health. It is great to do it every day.

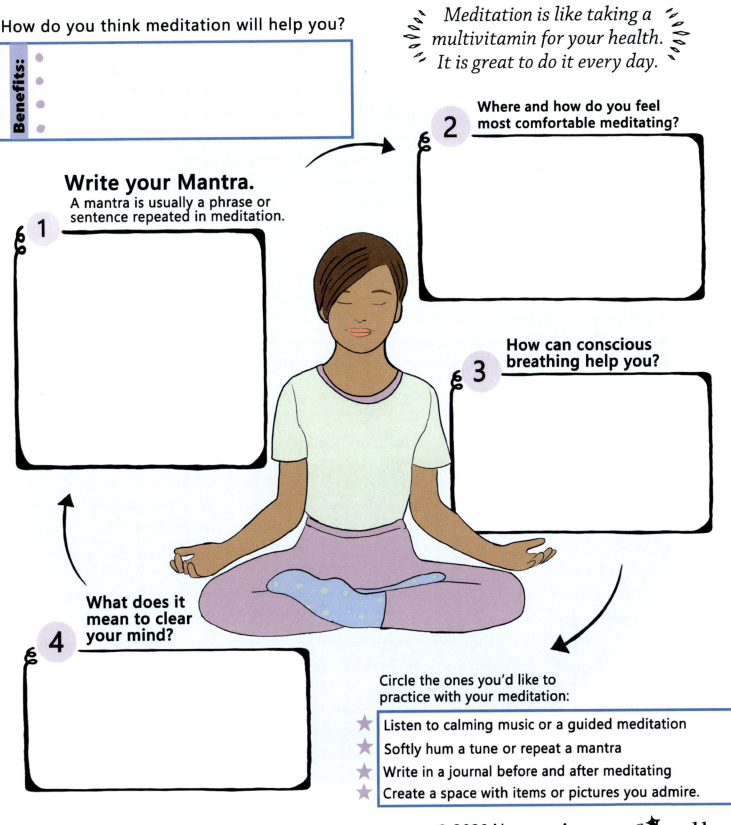

2 Where and how do you feel most comfortable meditating?

Write your Mantra.
A mantra is usually a phrase or sentence repeated in meditation.

1

3 How can conscious breathing help you?

What does it mean to clear your mind?

4

Circle the ones you'd like to practice with your meditation:

★ Listen to calming music or a guided meditation

★ Softly hum a tune or repeat a mantra

★ Write in a journal before and after meditating

★ Create a space with items or pictures you admire.

Name _____ Date___/___/_____

© 2020 Neurons Away

Self-Healing
Meditation

Help by sending magical energy to any parts of your body that do not feel well.

1 IMAGINE A GLOWING LIGHT ABOVE YOUR HEAD.

2 IMAGINE THE LIGHT TOUCHING YOUR HEAD AND FLOWING OVER YOUR BODY.

3 AS YOU BREATHE FEEL THE LIGHT COME IN THROUGH YOUR NOSE.

4 FEEL THE LIGHT GO DOWN INTO YOUR CHEST AND THROUGH YOUR ARMS AND SHOOT OUT OF YOUR FINGER TIPS.

5 FEEL THE LIGHT GO DOWN YOUR BELLY, THROUGH YOUR LEGS, AND COME OUT OF THE TIPS OF YOUR TOES.

Your body has the wonderful ability to heal itself.

Name _____ Date ___/___/_____

Can you draw or explain what healing energy might feel or look like?

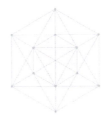

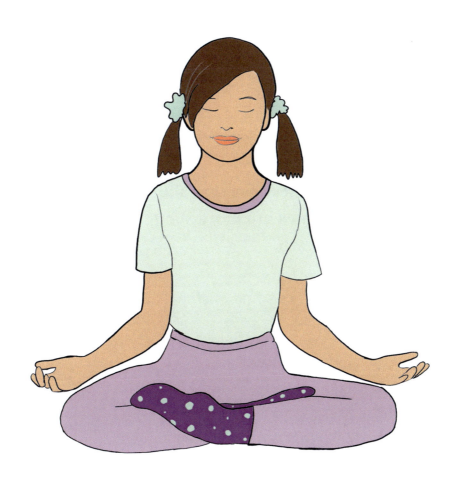

Self-Awareness

Self-awareness is about learning to understand your thoughts and feelings and how they may effect your actions and behavior.

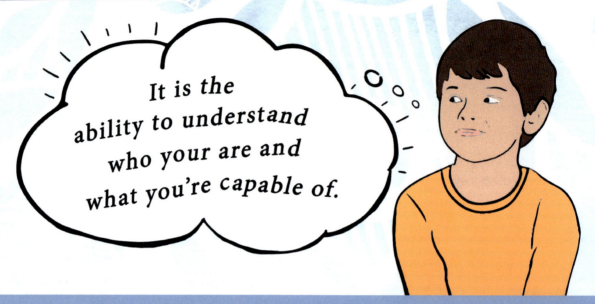

It is *the* ability to understand who your are and what you're *capable of.*

WAYS TO PRACTICE SELF AWARENESS:

Learn your thoughts and emotions

How:

Notice your thoughts and feelings throughout the day. You can do this by keeping a journal or by spend 5-10 minutes thinking about how your day went.

★ Did you yell because things didn't go your way?

★ Did you stay calm and use your words?

Ask yourself the right questions

How:

Ask questions that allow you to learn more about yourself.

Here are some examples:

★ What is good for me and my growth?

★ Who do I want to become?

★ What can I do to help myself?

Understand your values

How:

Identify what is most important to you and how you want to spend your time.

★ Do you want to improve in a certain sport or activity?

★ Do you want to be a kind and responsible friend?

★ Do you want to be more creative?

Name _____ Date___/___/____ © 2020 Neurons Away 14

Building Your Character

As you grow, who do you want to become?

Learning to be your own person can be challenging and full of surprises.
We tend to learn from the people and enviroment around us.

Different ways to understand and build your character:

Surround yourself with positive influences.

Choose friends, teachers, videos, and other things that have a positive influence on your life and choices.

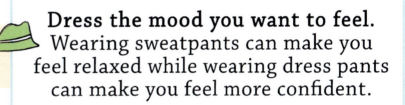

Change up your style

Dress the mood you want to feel. Wearing sweatpants can make you feel relaxed while wearing dress pants can make you feel more confident.

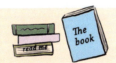

Read fiction.

Reading stories can help expand your understanding of life. Stories can show you different perspectives and personalities that may influence you in positive ways.

Try new activities.

Trying new activities will let you learn your own abilities and help you build on a variety of skills.

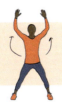

Exercise

Body movement is a great way to keep your character strong and your body and mind healthy.

Do you see yourself for who you really are?

Understand yourself by asking the right questions

What's most important to you?

What makes you happy?

What influences your behavior?

What are your strengths?

What are weaknesses you want to improve upon?

How can you get to know yourself more?

What do you see in your reflection?

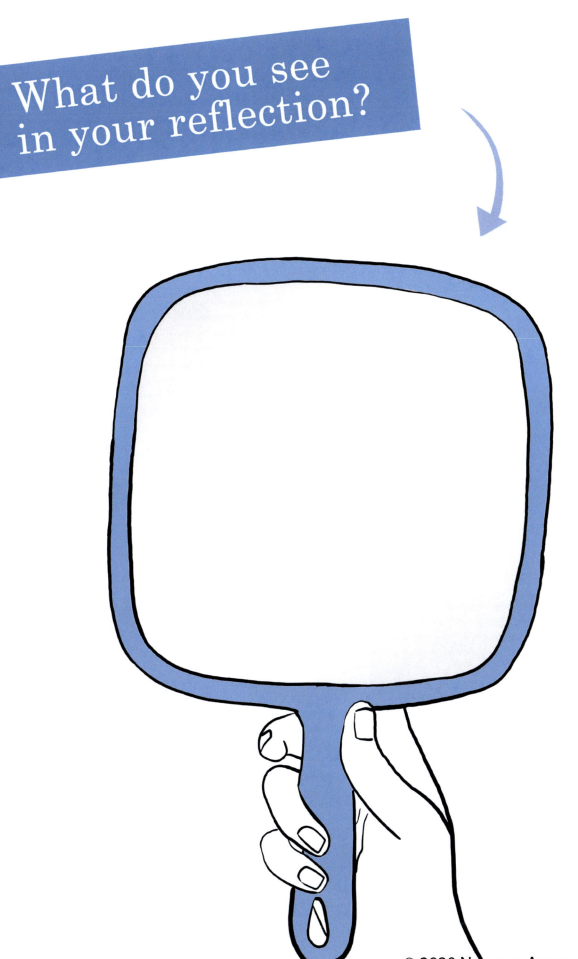

Healthy Socializing

Interacting with others in a friendly way

Socializing means:

- **Making new friends**
- **Having fun with others**
- **Sharings similar interests**
- **Joining groups & activities**
- **Learning with others**

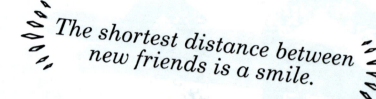

The shortest distance between new friends is a smile.

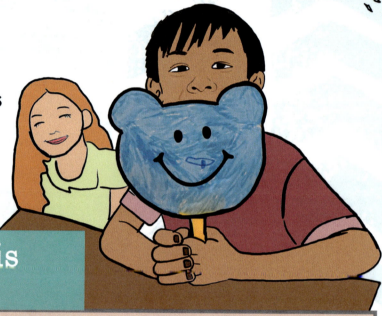

Healthy socializing is important because...

→ It helps develop self-confidence and communciations skills

→ It is a part of building meaningful friendships

→ It is a helpful way to learn about the world and other people

Ways to build healthy social connections:

* Take a walk with a friend
* Play a game or read with others
* Teach someone a skill you may know
* Ask someone to teach you a skill
* Introduce yourself to someone new

* Join an activity group
* Make something together
* Help out someone in need
* Ask a new kid to play with you
* Write a story with someone

Name_____ Date___/___/___

The ⑤ people you spend the most time with help shape who you are.

We are influenced by the people closest to us. They affect our way of thinking, our self-image, and our decision making. Of course, everyone is their own person, but sometimes we are influenced by our surrounding in more ways than we may understand.

1. List 5 ways you could improve your relationships with friends or family.

_____

_____

_____

_____

2. List 5 different groups or activities you want to join.

_____

_____

_____

_____

3. List 5 personality traits you are looking for in a new friend.

_____

_____

_____

_____

4. List 5 ways you can change an unhealthy social environment.

_____

_____

_____

_____

_____

5. List 5 positive traits you want to gain from the people that surround you.

Name _____ Date___/___/_____

Conversation Starters:

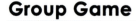

Sitting with some friends or a new group of people?
Try sparking a conversation with one of the questions below:

Group Game

1. Begin by letting one person choose a question.
2. Going in a circle, let each person respond.
   (the person who chose the questions goes last)
3. Each player must provide a response within a total time of 3 minutes.
   (3 minutes for the entire group NOT each person)
4. If the group goes over 3 minutes the person who chose the question gets to make a rule.
   (example: raise both arms while talking)
5. For each round completed within 3 mins the group gets 5 points. *(adjust time if necessary)*

1. What is your favorite food?

2. What's your favorite season? Why?

3. Where do good thoughts and ideas come from?

4. What would it feel like to be a tree?

5. What are three things you want to learn?

Add some new questions to the list.

6. Where is the most beautiful place near where you live?

7. What do you do to improve your mood when you are in a bad mood?

8. What do you have that you are grateful for?

9. What would life be like if there was no such thing as sound?

10. What are the good things in life?

11. What are the ways you can make someone smile?

12. Where does happiness come from?

13. What are three things the world needs more of?

14. What's the coolest thing you've ever seen?

15. What makes a good friendship?

16. What are some of your favorite movies?

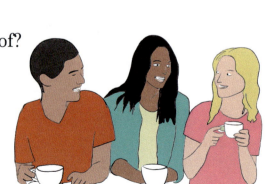

Name _____ Date___/___/_____   © 2020 Neurons Away   20

Circle the activities you would like to try and place a star next your top three choices.

To lead a fulfilling and happy life it is important to stay engaged and active in the community. Joining new classes, involving yourself in new activities and staying physically active can change and improve the dynamics of your lifestyle.

Things to do just for fun

1. Kite Flying
2. Trip to the Museum
3. Visit a second-hand shop
4. Trip to an Art Gallery
5. Attend a theatre show
6. Trip to an amusement park
7. Attend a concert
8. Visit a zoo or animal shelter
9. Spend the day at the beach
10. Go see a movie
11. Volunteer
12. Read
13. Write a short book
14. Take day trip
15. Skip rocks
16. Sudoku
17. Crossword puzzles
18. Word searches
19. Chess
20. Checkers
21. Scrabble
22. Card games
23. Create card pyramids
24. Dominoes
25. Bingo
26. Learn to meditate
27. Nature walk/hike
28. Visit a café
29. Part time job/volunteer
30. Explore your city

Team Sports

31. Hockey
32. Soccer
33. Basketball
34. Baseball
35. Football
36. Volleyball
37. Rugby
38. Ultimate Frisbee
39. Lacrosse
40. Tennis
41. Bowling
42. Fencing
43. Golf
44. Synchronized swimming

Sports/Activities

45. Swimming
46. Running/Jogging
47. Kayaking
48. Martial Arts
49. Biking
50. Canoeing
51. Rock Climbing
52. Snowboarding
53. Skiing
54. Surfing
55. Skating
56. Roller blading
57. Calisthenics
58. Archery
59. Fishing
60. Gymnastics
61. Yoga
62. Acrobatics
63. Pilates
64. Tai Chi
65. Hiking
66. Horseback riding
67. Juggling
68. Scuba diving
69. Snorkeling
70. Weight lifting
71. Tread mill

Dance

72. Irish dancing
73. Salsa dancing
74. Hip hop
75. Tap
76. Swing
77. Belly-dancing
78. Ballet
79. Break-dancing
80. Zumba

Creative Hobbies

81. Cooking/Baking
82. Cake Making / Decorating
83. Sculpting
84. Furniture building
85. Woodcarving
86. Flower arranging
87. Coloring
88. Watercolor painting
89. Oil painting
90. Glass painting
91. Chalk drawing
92. Rapping/Free styling
93. Collecting (e.g. stamps)
94. Origami
95. Calligraphy
96. Jewelry making
97. Gardening
98. Magic tricks
99. Photography
100. Writing
101. Poetry writing
102. Sewing
103. Knitting
104. Embroidery
105. Making dream-catchers
106. Weaving (baskets, etc)
107. Scrap-booking
108. Learn to play a musical instrument. (guitar, flute)
109. Learn a new language
110. Restoration/refurbishing
111. Canning/jarring

5-4-3-2-1-Relax

Engage your 5 senses to help you reconnect and feel calmer in the present moment.

Look around you and **find 5** of each: 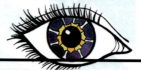 **SIGHT**

Five circular shapes	Five tiny items	Five blue objects
		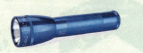

TOUCH — Feel with your hands

Find & feel 4 items for 20 seconds each
1. a hard and sturdy item
2. a soft or fluffy item
3. a flexible and bendy item
4. a rough or bumpy item

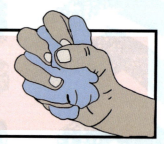

HEARING — Listen to your surroundings

Identify 3 different sounds
1. listen to the sounds close to you
2. listen for background sounds
3. listen to the sound of your breath

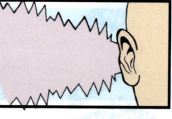

SMELL — Engage your nose

Sniff out 2 scents from your surrounding
1. a scent that you enjoy (flowers, soap, bread, etc.)
2. a strong scent that stimulates your nose (coffee, lotion, etc.)

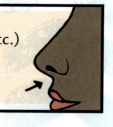

TASTE — On the tip of your tongue

Engage your taste buds by trying 1 of each: Something **Sweet,** something **Sour** and something **Salty.**

   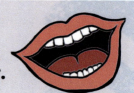

Name _____ Date___/___/_____   © 2020 Neurons Away   22

5-4-3-2-1-Relax

Engage your 5 senses to help you reconnect and feel calmer in the present moment.

5 **Observe your surroundings and identify 5 of the following:**

Circular objects	Tiny items	Blue items
_____	_____	_____
_____	_____	_____
_____	_____	_____
_____	_____	_____
_____	_____	_____

4 **Find and feel 4 items -** *touch or hold for 10 seconds each*

a hard item   a soft item   a flexible item   a smooth item

_____   _____   _____   _____

3 **Listen to your surroundings and identify 3 different sounds:**

2 **Engage your nose by sniffing out 2 different smells**
Seek out scents you enjoy such as flowers, soap, lotion etc.

1 **On the tip of your tongue try tasting one of the following**
OR find and try them all! (If you don't have access to food at the moment use your imagination. Imagine biting into a lemon or sprinkling salt on your tongue.)

Sweet   **Sour**   and **Salty**

YOUR SELF-TALK

Self-talk is the voice inside of you that helps you understand yourself and the world around you.

1 *Listen to what you're saying to yourself.*

→ Where are these thoughts and words coming from?

→ Are they words you learned from others?

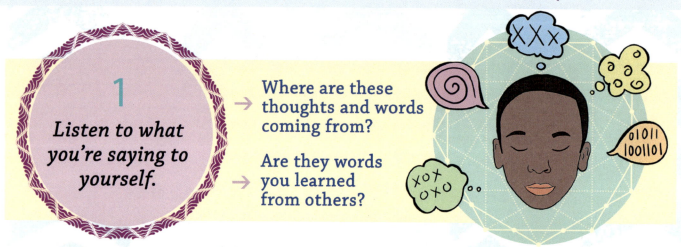

2 *Is your self-talk helping you or not helping you?*

→ How are your thoughts and words making you feel?

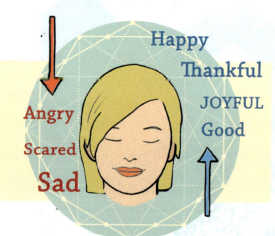

Angry
Scared
Sad

Happy
Thankful
JOYFUL
Good

3 *How can you change your self-talk to make you feel better?*

→ What are some nice things you can tell yourself?

→ What words can you use to help your mood?

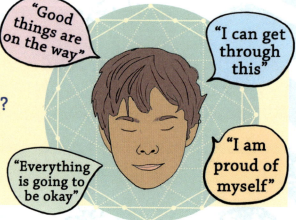

"Good things are on the way"

"I can get through this"

"Everything is going to be okay"

"I am proud of myself"

The Art of Self Talk

Use this worksheet to learn more about your inner dialogue

What is self-talk? It's the voice in your head that narrates your life and perspective. Sometimes it can have a negative or positive impact on your emotions.

If in a group setting:
-Discuss where different kinds of self-talk come from.
-How it can affect your mindset and well-being.
-Share examples of healthy self-talk.

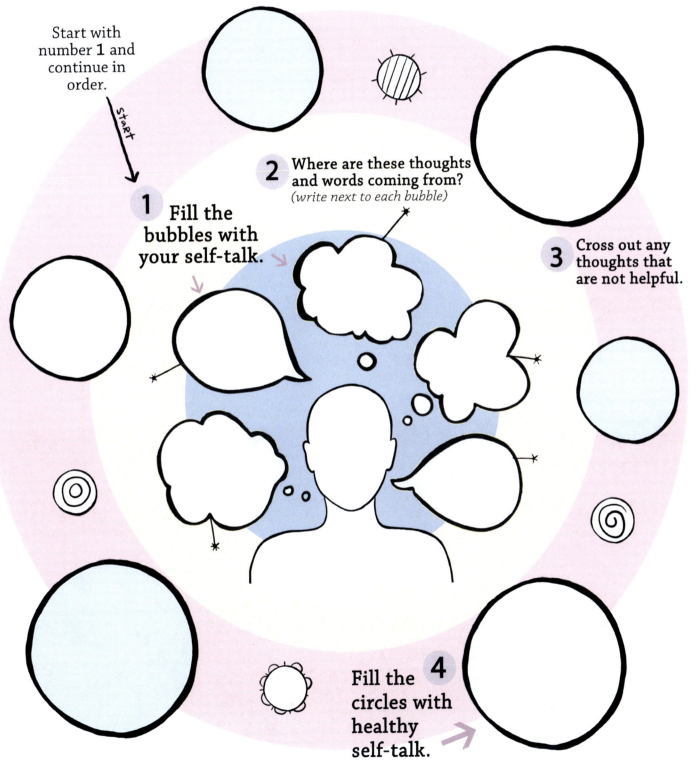

Start with number **1** and continue in order.

START

1 Fill the bubbles with your self-talk.

2 Where are these thoughts and words coming from? *(write next to each bubble)*

3 Cross out any thoughts that are not helpful.

4 Fill the circles with healthy self-talk.

USE YOUR HANDS

To reduce stress when dealing with a difficult situation.

START SMALL & SIMPLE

1- Hold an ice cube

Find an ice cube and hold it in your hand for as long as you can! Give the ice cube your attention and notice the feeling.

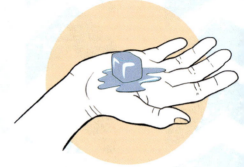

2- Wash your hands in warm water

Warm water can calm you down.
When feeling very stressed wash your hands under warm water for 1 minute. Feel the water cleaning your emotions from your hands.

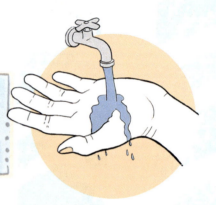

3 - Squeeze a rubber ball

Squeeze the ball for a few seconds and then release. As your muscles relax, the tension will leave your arms and hands, taking away stress.

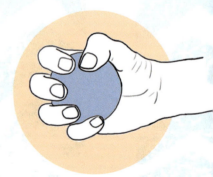

4 - Squish playdough

Squishing playdough through your fingers can release frustration and anger. As you squeze through the play dough make different shapes to express your creativity.

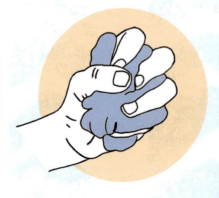

Name _____ Date___/___/_____

USE YOUR HANDS

Using a stress ball can help redirect your mind away from stress and help you to relax

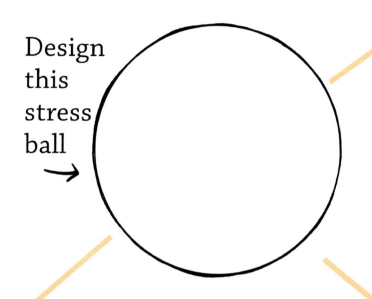

Design
this
stress
ball →

Squeeze a rubber ball

1- Hold the ball in your hand notice the weight and texture.

2- Squeeze the ball as tight as possible for 5 seconds.

3- Release your grip for 5 seconds

4- Repeat 10 times.

When you are experiencing high stress or overwhelming emotions, your body is holding a lot of unhealthy energy and it has no where to go.
A physical release is a helpful way to let go of that unhealthy energy.

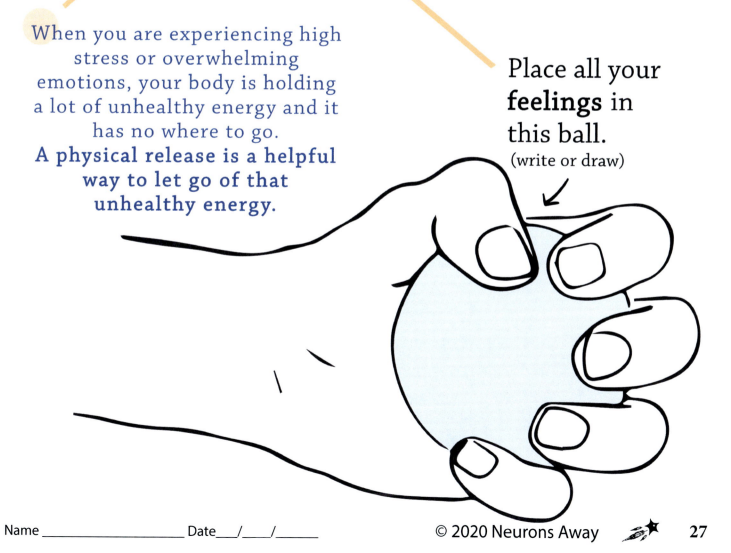

Place all your
feelings in
this ball.
(write or draw)

Wash your hands in warm water

Warm water immediately engages a calming response.

In the moment of a stressful event, removing yourself to wash your hands can give you both the space and body connection to regain composure.

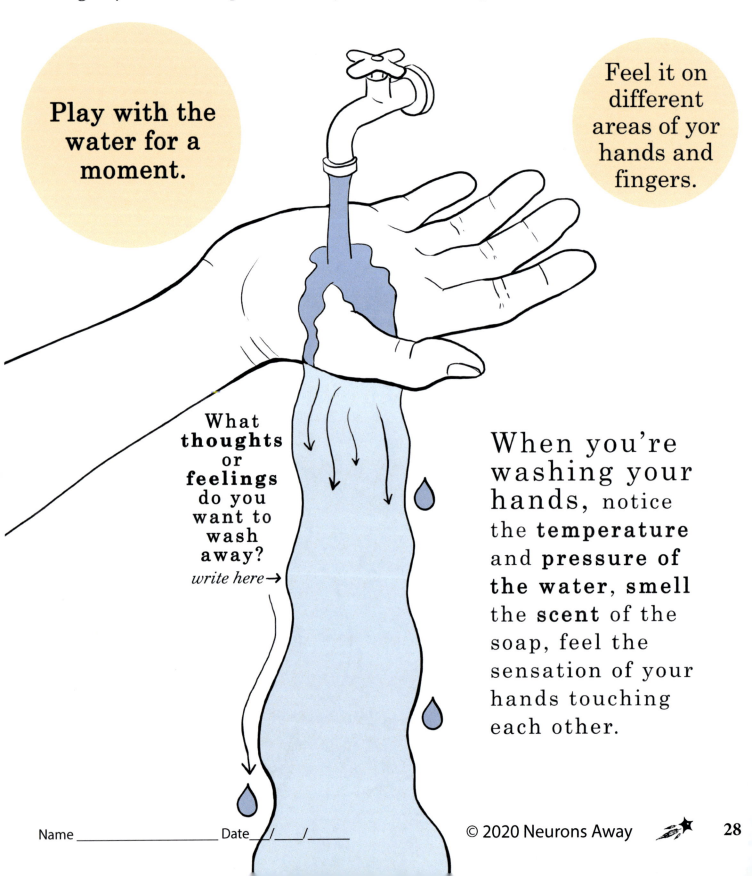

Play with the water for a moment.

Feel it on different areas of yor hands and fingers.

What thoughts or feelings do you want to wash away?

write here →

When you're washing your hands, notice the **temperature** and **pressure of the water, smell** the **scent** of the soap, feel the sensation of your hands touching each other.

Movement is Medicine

Moving your body can help create positive changes with your emotions and thoughts.

Exercising your core can make you feel **strong**, **balanced** and **confident.**

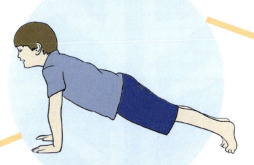

Hold a plank for 1 minute or Attempt to do 5 push-ups 2 times.

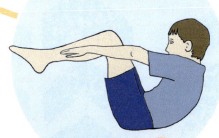

Do 10 sit ups or Kick your feet like you are riding a bicycle for 1 minute

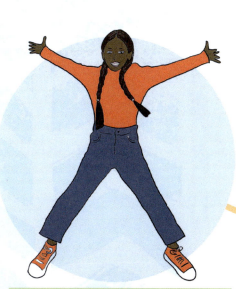

Do 20 jumping jacks 2 times or Hold your hands high in the air for 1 minute

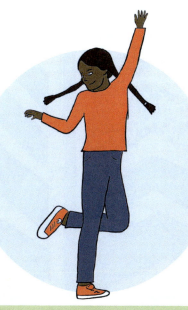

Dance for 2 or more minutes or Run in place for 1 minute

Moving your body in different ways can **boost your mood** and **lessen stress.**

Movement is Medicine

Moving your body can help create positive changes with your emotions or thoughts.

COLOR AND PLAY

1. Choose an exercise from the page to do.
2. After you perform the exercises color in the figure you chose
3. Continue until all figures are colored in.

IF PLAYING IN A GROUP

1. Choose an exercise (a or b) for everyone in the group to complete.
2. Color the figure in after the exercises has been completed.
3. Continue until all figures are fully colored in.
(for an extra challenge complete both a & b exercises)

2

a - Hold a plank for 30 seconds

or   b - Attempt to do 5 pushups

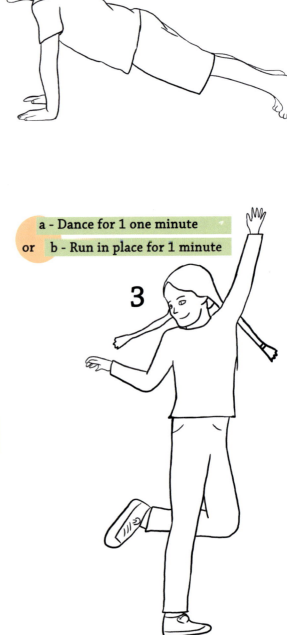

1

a - Do 20 jumping jacks

or   b - Hold your hands high in the air for 1

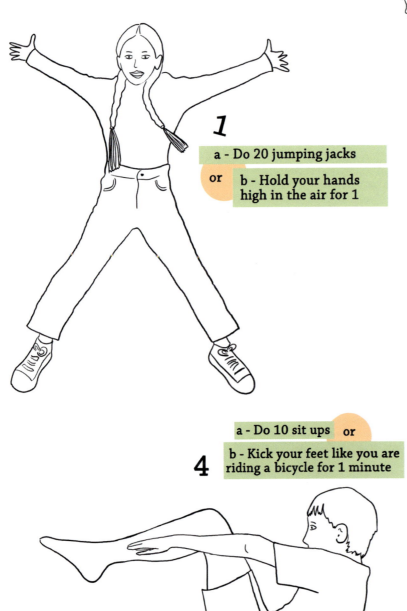

a - Dance for 1 one minute

or   b - Run in place for 1 minute

3

a - Do 10 sit ups   or

b - Kick your feet like you are riding a bicycle for 1 minute

4

Name _____ Date___/____/_____

30

Movement is Medicine

Moving Your Body Is Good for Your Mind

Exercise releases endorphins, which create feelings of happiness and helps boost self-esteem and confidence.

Seated Jacks

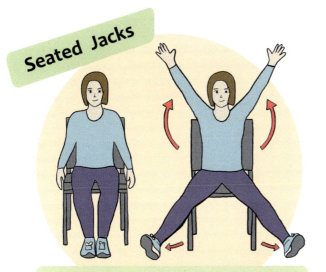

1 Start at the edge of your seat, knees bent and arms at your side.

2 Then at the same time raise your arms and extend your legs wide to the sides Bring arms and legs back to center.

3 Repeat 20 times.

Seated Twists

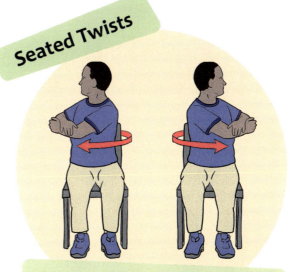

1 Fold your arms in front of you.

2 Turn your upper body to the side let your head follow last.

3 Twist to the other side. Go slow and repeat this 20 times.

Leg Extensions

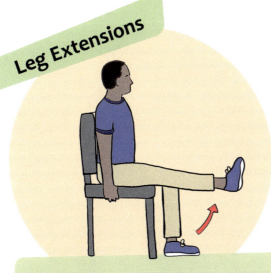

1 Hold the side of your chair for support. Lift and extend one leg in front of you.

2 Then lift the other leg. Repeat on each side 10 times.

Peekaboo

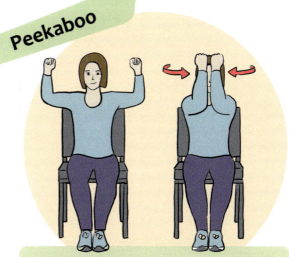

1 Hold your arms up to the side with elbows bent and palms facing forward.

2 Bring your forearms together in front of your face. Repeat 20 times.

Name _____ Date___/___/_____

Movement is Medicine (Seated Exercises)

Various forms of exercises can boost your mood, ease depression and anxiety enhance your self-esteem, and improve your whole outlook on life.

COLOR AND PLAY

1. Choose an exercise from the page to do.
2. After you perform the exercises color in the figure you chose
3. Contiune until all figures are colored in.

IF PLAYING IN A GROUP

1. Choose an exercise for everyone in the group to complete.
2. Color the figure in after the exercises has been completed.
3. Contiune until all figures are fully colored in.

Seated Twists 3

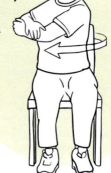

Twist your upper body from side to side. Repeat 10 times on each side.

March in Place

2 While seated march in place. Swing the opposite arm as you march each foot forward.

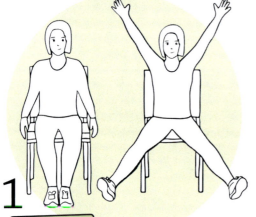

1

Seated Jacks

Raise your arms and extend your legs wide and to the sides. Repeat 20 times.

Peekaboo

4 Bring your forearms together in front of your face. Repeat 20 times.

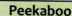
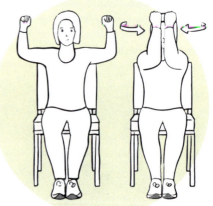

6 **Leg Extensions**

Lift and extend each leg up. Repeat on each leg 10 times.

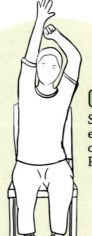
5

Arm Extensions

Stretch and reach each arm high over your head. Repeat 20 times.

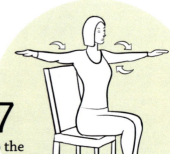

7

Leg Extensions

Extend your arms to the side. Rotate shoulders and arms 20 times forward and 20 times backwards.

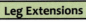
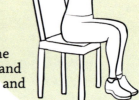
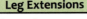

Name _____ Date___/___/_____

© 2020 Neurons Away 32

Mindful Walking
A quick and easy way to feel better.

Find a clear space where you can walk back and forth.

While standing **Move your weight from side to side and tap each foot gently against the floor.**

Take a deep breath, lift your head and look straight ahead with your chest held high.

Place your hands to your side or hold them behind your back.

Begin walking, step one foot

As you step forward notice how the other leg begins to lift up.

Count ten steps forward.

On your tenth step stop and **take a deep breath.**

Turn around and walk back to the other side continuing the same practice.

Do this for about 10 to 15 minutes or until you are feeling better.

Name_____ Date____/____/_____

UNWIND YOUR MIND
with this exercise

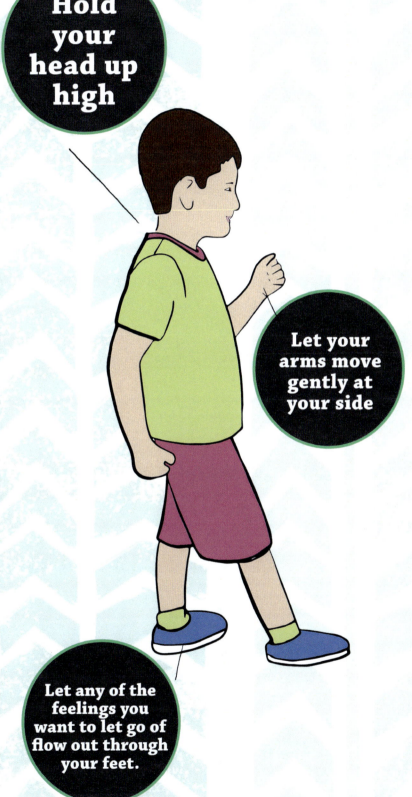

Hold your head up high

Let your arms move gently at your side

Let any of the feelings you want to let go of flow out through your feet.

Mindful Walking
A quick and easy way to feel better.

Find a clear space where you can walk back and forth.

While standing **Move your weight from side to side and tap each foot gently against the floor.**

Take a deep breath, lift your head and look straight ahead with your chest held high.

Place your hands to your side or hold them behind your back.

Begin walking, step one foot

As you step forward notice how the other leg begins to lift up.

Count ten steps forward.

On your tenth step stop and **take a deep breath.**

Turn around and walk back to the other side continuing the same practice.

Do this for about 10 to 15 minutes or until you are feeling better.

Before Walking:

How are you currently feeling?
(Write down at least three emotions)

_____

_____

_____

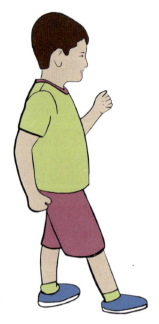

Circle where you feel these emotions:
(if they are emotions you wish to release, draw lines that release them through the feet)

How and **why** might mindful walking help you release unwanted feelings?

_____

_____

_____

After Walking:

How are you currently feeling?
(Write down at least three emotions)

_____

_____

_____

Draw one thing you remember from your walk:

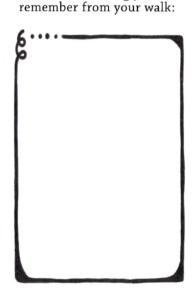

Do you feel a **difference?**

Yes / No

If yes explain why:

_____

_____

_____

If no explain why and what you might do differently next time:

_____

_____

_____

_____

_____

_____

_____

Mindful Walking

A great way to guide your emotions, calm the body, and focus the mind.

the ideal walk:

Use this page to plan out and guide your walks.

What thoughts do you want in your head?

Where do you want your legs to take you?

What do you want to gain from your walk?

What do energey or emotions do you want released into the ground?

Understanding Your Story

Creating a healthy story for yourself

What's your story?

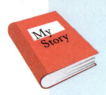
Your story is the narrative you identify yourself by. It's how you introduce yourself and interact with the world. Your story influences your perspective and decisions making.

How do these stories form?

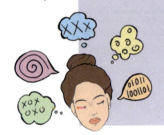
The stories we live by are influenced by our **past experiences,** by the **words and actions others show us** and by our **beliefs.** These influences can be negative, positive or neutral.

Identify what's helping and what's hindering.

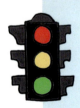
It's important to understand the stories and beliefs you hold close to you. Are they mental blocks or growth promoting thoughts? What part of your story makes you feel stuck? What part of your story inspires you?

Transforming the stories.

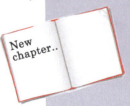
You might not be able to control the facts of your life, but you can control the way it influences you. You have the ability to change beliefs and thoughts. You have the ability to tell new stories.

Change Your Story

6 ways to improve your story:

Purpose:
New outlook on life
Creating change from within
Opens up new opportunities

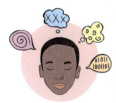

Use your imagination creatively
When you imagine yourself winning a game or doing something fun you can generate a feeling of confidence or excitement. However, if you use your mind to worry about failing a test or to hold bitter thoughts this can make you feel anxious or stressed.

Visualize yourself doing something very different
Imagine yourself climbing a big mountain, swimming in the ocean, or walking through a rain forest. What sounds do you hear, what scents do you smell, what colors do you see? Using your mind to explore new places can introduce you to new thoughts and feelings without having to go anywhere!

List all the different possible things you can be see and do!
Think about all the possible outcomes you can have. Write them down even if some are out of your comfort zone. List all possible jobs, studies, hobbies, places you'll visit, etc. This will help you learn more about you and your interests.

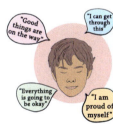

Use helpful self-talk
If you want change your story it's best to start with how you talk to yourself. For example, if you normally start the day by saying "I'm not a morning person." instead try saying, "I'm learning to like all parts the day, even the morning."

Write an inspiring story about yourself
You can use experiences from the past or dive deep into your imagination. Either way write a story that lifts your spirits and makes you smile. "I invented a cool new toy!" or "I finally got to see my favorite animal up close!"

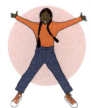

Keep play in your life.
Playing with friends, family and pets is a great way to improve problem-solving abilities and enhance emotional well-being. Plus it brings more joy into your life!

Name _____ Date____/____/_____

List all of the possible outcomes for yourself

Has anyone ever asked you: "What do you want to be when you grow up?" This is common question you might hear but it can sometimes be hard to answer. Sometimes you don't know exactly what you want to be, or there are many things you want to be!

Use this page to write down all the things you would like to be or do as you grow through life. Think of what jobs or careers you might have, what things you want to study in school or what lifestyles you want to try.

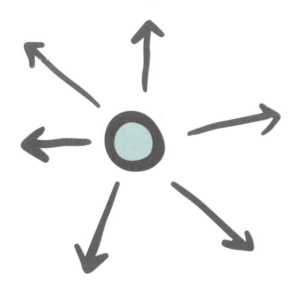

Write an inspiring story about yourself

You can use experiences from the past or dive deep into your imagination.
Either way write a story that lifts your spirits and makes you smile.
"I invented a cool new toy!" or "I finally got to see my favorite animal up close!"

Creating Your Life

How do you imagine your ideal life?
What is it filled with and what do you do?

Fill in bubbles with what you want your life to be filled with.

Emotions / Mindsets

Skills / Hobbies

Friendships

Future Achievements

Future Job / Career

Things / Places

Acts of Self Care

Self-care is process of treating yourself well.
This includes taking care of your body and mind.

CHOOSE 3 OF YOUR FAVORITE ACTIVITIES TO DO TODAY

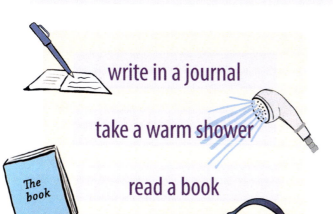

write in a journal

take a warm shower

read a book

sing or listen to music

write a song or poetry

eat a healthy snack

drink lots of water

write a nice letter to yourself

create a vision board

say nice things to yourself

Create yourself a new schedule

do some exercises

list everything you are proud of

meditate or relax

stretch your body out

massage your head and neck

rub lotion on your hands

Take deep breaths

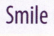

Brush your teeth

Smile

It is important to give yourself time and space to include self-beneficial activities throughout your week.

"The way you treat yourself sets the standard for others."

The Importance of Self Care

Self-care is about doing things that improve your quality of life.
This includes emotional, physical and spiritual wellbeing

List the ways you can care for yourself

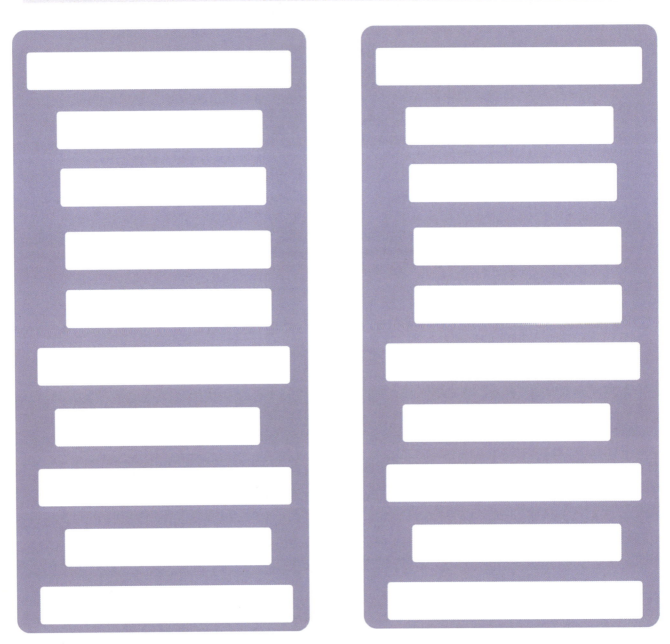

It is important to give yourself time and space to include
self-beneficial activities throughout your week.

"The way you treat yourself sets the standard for others."

Name _____ Date___/___/_____

Distract Yourself in Healthy Ways

Perhaps the simplest way to calm your mind is to distract yourself by focusing on some other thought, interest, or activity that holds and redirects your attention.

CHOOSE 3 TO DO TODAY

- ☐ Learn to juggle
- ☐ Doodle or draw
- ☐ Plan a journey
- ☐ Listen to music
- ☐ Floss your teeth
- ☐ Eat a piece of fruit
- ☐ Learn to moonwalk
- ☐ Daydream
- ☐ Squeeze your pillow
- ☐ Take a nap
- ☐ Memorize a poem
- ☐ Learn origami
- ☐ Draw a self portrait
- ☐ Write a bucket list
- ☐ Play solitaire

- ☐ Make up some jokes
- ☐ Draw your favorite room
- ☐ Leave nice notes in random places
- ☐ Learn about a new culture
- ☐ Celebrate a small success
- ☐ Make up a new smoothie recipe
- ☐ Write a list of fun things to do
- ☐ Learn or make up a new song
- ☐ Clean/reorganize your space
- ☐ Give yourself a foot massage
- ☐ Write a letter to a friend
- ☐ Watch a new movie or TV show
- ☐ Share a funny story
- ☐ Draw the cover to your book
- ☐ Write a list of your achievements

Name _____ Date ___/___/_____

PRACTICE GOOD HYGIENE
(Hi-Jeen)

Use these methods to stay healthy and prevent disease.

1 wash your hands

Lather your hands with soap and water for 20 seconds.

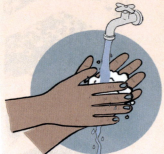

1. Wet Hands
2. Add soap
3. Scrub your hands and _under your nails_ (While singing the ABCs)
3. Rinse your hands
4. Dry Hands

IMPORTANT TIMES TO WASH
- Before and after eating
- After school
- After going out in public
- After using the bathroom
- Before going to sleep

2 Respect Personal Space

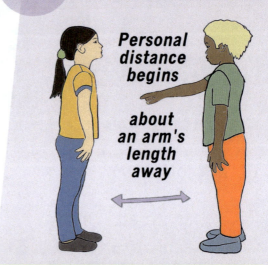

Personal distance begins

about an arm's length away

- Don't breathe on others
- Keep your hands to yourself

3 Don't touch your face

Germs enter through eyes, nose and mouth.

- Avoid rubbing your eyes
- Wipe your nose with a tissue
NOT on your sleeve or hand

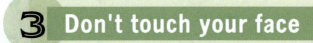

Keep your fingers **AWAY** from your mouth

4 Cover Your Cough or Sneeze

Germs can travel up to 6 feet.

Sneeze Into Your **Elbow**, Not Your Hand.

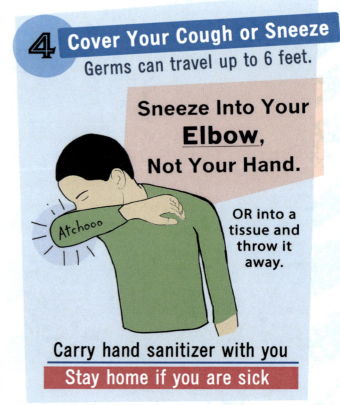

Atchooo

OR into a tissue and throw it away.

Carry hand sanitizer with you

Stay home if you are sick

© 2020 Neurons Away

PRACTICE GOOD HYGIENE
(Hi-Jeen)

List four other ways you can stay healthy and prevent the spread of germs.

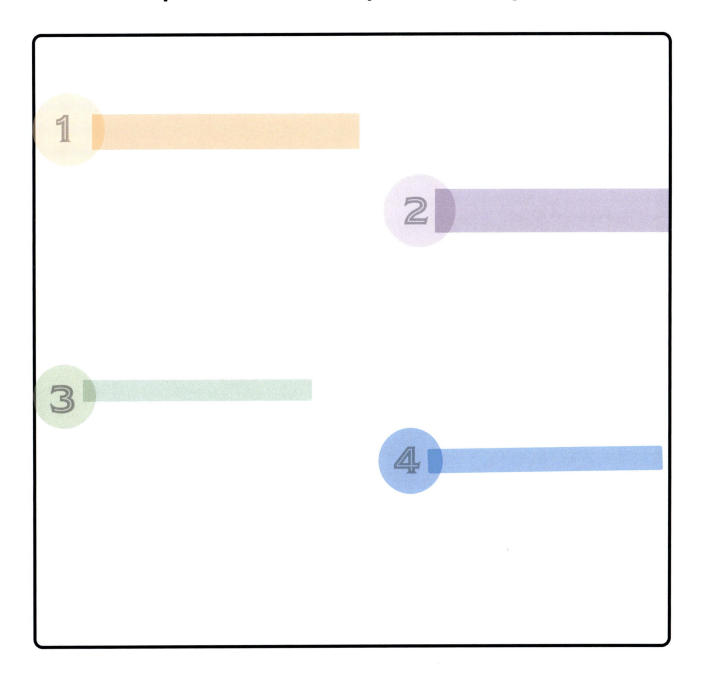

1

2

3

4

A vision board is collection of images, pictures and affirmations of interests and desires, designed to serve as a source of inspiration and motivation.

My Faith

Things that make me happy.

Places I want to travel.

My goals in life.

Things I am grateful for.

Things I want to learn.

Love and friendship ♥ ♥

Name_____ Date___/___/____

Made in the USA
Middletown, DE
13 July 2021

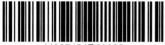